The Hormone Reset Diet:

10+1 Hormone Diet Strategies with First Results in Just 10 Days

John J. Filler

Hormones and Obesity

What is obesity?

Obesity is a scourge in the United States. This condition puts individuals at a higher hazard for genuine infections, for example, type 2 diabetes, coronary illness, and malignant growth. As per the Centers for Disease Control and Prevention (CDC), it's assessed that in 2015–2016, 93.3 million American grown-ups and 13.7 million American youngsters and teenagers are clinically corpulent. Weight is characterized as having a weight list (BMI) of at least 30. BMI is an estimation that considers an individual's weight and stature. In any case, BMI has a few impediments. As indicated by the CDCTrusted Source, "Factors, for example, age, sex, ethnicity, and bulk can impact the connection among BMI and muscle to fat ratio. Additionally, BMI doesn't recognize overabundance fat, muscle, or bone mass, nor does it give any sign of the circulation of fat among people."

In spite of these impediments, BMI keeps on being generally utilized as a marker of overabundance weight.

What causes obesity?

Eating a obeser number of calories than you consume in day by day action and exercise (on a drawn out premise) causes obesity. After some time, these additional calories include and cause you to put on weight.Normal explicit reasons for obesity include:

- eating a horrible eating routine of foods high in fats and calories
- having a stationary (inert) way of life

- not resting enough, which can prompt hormonal changes that cause you to feel hungrier and long for certain unhealthy foods
- hereditary qualities, which can influence how your body forms food into vitality and how fat is put away
- developing more established, which can prompt less bulk and a more slow metabolic rate, making it simpler to put on weight
- pregnancy (weight picked up during pregnancy can be hard to lose and may in the end lead to obesity)
- Certain ailments may likewise prompt weight gain. These include:
- polycystic ovary disorder (PCOS): a condition that causes an irregularity of female conceptive hormones

- Prader-Willi disorder: an uncommon condition that an individual is brought into the world with which causes unreasonable appetite
- Cushing disorder: a condition brought about by having an over the top measure of the hormone cortisol in your framework
- hypothyroidism (underactive thyroid): a condition where the thyroid organ doesn't deliver enough of certain significant hormones
- osteoarthritis (and different conditions that cause torment that may prompt idleness.)

Who is at risk for obesity?

A mind boggling blend of hereditary, natural, and mental elements can build an individual's hazard for obesity.

Genetics

A few people have hereditary elements that make it hard for them to get in shape.

Environment and community

Your condition at home, at school, and in your locale, would all be able to impact how and what you eat and how dynamic you are. Perhaps you haven't figured out how to prepare solid dinners or don't figure you can manage the cost of more advantageous foods. In the event that your neighborhood is risky, possibly you haven't found a decent spot to play, walk, or run.

Psychological and other factors

Wretchedness can once in a while lead to weight gain, as individuals go to food for enthusiastic solace. Certain antidepressants can likewise build danger of weight gain. It really is ideal to stop smoking, yet stopping can likewise prompt weight gain. Therefore, it's critical to concentrate on diet and exercise while you're stopping. Prescriptions, for example, steroids or contraception pills can likewise put you at more serious hazard for weight gain.

How is obesity Diagnosed?

Obesity is characterized as having a BMI of at least 30. Weight file is an unpleasant estimation of an individual's load comparable to their tallness.

Other progressively precise proportions of muscle to fat ratio and muscle to fat ratio dispersion incorporate skinfold thickness, midsection to-hip correlations, and screening tests, for example, ultrasound, processed tomography (CT), and attractive reverberation imaging (MRI) filters. Your primary care physician may likewise arrange certain tests to help analyze obesity just as obesity related wellbeing dangers. These may incorporate blood tests to inspect cholesterol and glucose levels, liver capacity tests, diabetes screen, thyroid tests, and heart tests, for example, an electrocardiogram.

An estimation of the fat around your midriff is likewise a decent indicator of hazard for obesity related ailments.

What are Complications of obesity?

Obesity prompts considerably more than straightforward weight gain. Having a high proportion of muscle versus fat to muscle puts strain on your bones just as your inner organs. It additionally builds irritation in the body, which is believed to be a reason for malignant growth. Obesity is additionally a significant reason for type 2 diabetes. Obesity has been connected to various wellbeing difficulties, some of which are perilous:

- type 2 diabetes
- coronary illness
- hypertension
- certain tumors (bosom, colon, and endometrial)
- stroke
- gallbladder malady
- greasy liver malady
- elevated cholesterol
- rest apnea and other breathing issues
- joint pain
- barrenness

How is obesity treated?

In case you're fat and haven't had the option to get in shape all alone, clinical assistance is accessible. Start with your family doctor who might have the option to allude you to a weight pro in your general vicinity. Your PCP may likewise need to work with you as a major aspect of a group helping you get more fit. That group may incorporate a dietitian, specialist, or potentially other medicinal services staff. Your PCP will work with you on making way of life changes. Here and there, they may suggest drugs or weight reduction medical procedure also.

Lifestyle and behavior changes

Your human services group can instruct you on better food decisions and help build up a good dieting arrangement that works for you. An organized exercise program and expanded day by day action — as long as 300 minutes per week — will help develop your quality, continuance, and digestion. Directing or bolster gatherings may likewise recognize undesirable triggers and assist you with adapting to any tension, despondency, or passionate eating issues.

Medical weight loss

Your primary care physician may likewise recommend certain medicine weight reduction meds notwithstanding smart dieting and exercise plans. Drugs are typically endorsed just if different techniques for weight reduction haven't worked and in the event that you have a BMI of at least 27 notwithstanding obesity related medical problems.

Remedy weight reduction meds either forestall the assimilation of fat or smother hunger. These medications can have upsetting reactions. For instance, the medication orlistat (Xenical) can prompt slick and continuous solid discharges, inside criticalness, and gas. Your primary care physician will screen you intently while you're taking these meds.

Weight loss surgery

Weight reduction medical procedure (regularly called "bariatric medical procedure") requires a responsibility from patients that they will change their way of life. These kinds of medical procedure work by constraining how much food you can easily eat or by keeping your body from engrossing food and calories. Now and again the two of them do. Weight reduction medical procedure is certainly not a handy solution. It's a significant medical procedure and can have genuine dangers. After medical procedure, patients should change how they eat and the amount they eat or chance becoming ill. Possibility for weight reduction medical procedure will have a BMI of at least 40, or have a BMI of 35 to 39.9 alongside genuine obesity related medical issues. Patients will regularly need to get in shape preceding experiencing medical procedure. Moreover, they will regularly experience advising to guarantee that they're both sincerely arranged for this medical procedure and ready to make the vital way of life changes that it will require.

Surgical options include:

- gastric detour medical procedure, which makes a little pocket at the head of your stomach that associates legitimately to your small digestive system. Food and fluids experience the pocket and into the digestive tract, bypassing a obese portion of the stomach.
- laparoscopic movable gastric banding (LAGB), which isolates your stomach into two pockets utilizing a band

- gastric sleeve, which evacuates some portion of your stomach
- biliopancreatic redirection with duodenal switch, which expels the greater part of your stomach

What is the long-term outlook for obesity?

There's been an emotional increment in weight and in obesity related maladies. This is the motivation behind why networks, states, and the government are putting an accentuation on solid food decisions and exercises to help reverse the situation on obesity. At last, be that as it may, the duty is on every one of us to roll out these solid improvements.

How can you prevent obesity?

Help forestall weight gain by settling on great way of life decisions. Focus on moderate exercise (strolling, swimming, biking) for 20 to 30 minutes consistently. Eat well by picking nutritious foods like natural products, vegetables, entire grains, and lean protein. Eat high-fat, fatty foods with some restraint.

Hormones are synthetic delivery people that direct procedures in our body. They are one factor in causing obesity. The hormones leptin and insulin, sex hormones and growth hormone impact our craving, digestion (the rate at which our body consumes kilojoules for vitality), and muscle to fat ratio dissemination. Individuals who are obese have levels of these hormones that support anomalous digestion and the collection of muscle to fat ratio. An arrangement of organs, known as the endocrine framework, secretes hormones into our circulatory system. The endocrine framework works with the sensory system and the safe framework to enable our body to adapt to various occasions and stresses. Abundances or shortages of hormones can prompt obesity and, then again, weight can prompt changes in hormones.

Obesity and leptin

The hormone leptin is delivered by fat cells and is emitted into our circulatory system. Leptin diminishes an individual's craving by following up on explicit focuses of their brain to decrease their desire to eat. It additionally appears to control how the body deals with its store of muscle versus fat.

Since leptin is created by fat, leptin levels will in general be higher in individuals who are corpulent than in individuals of ordinary weight. Notwithstanding, regardless of having more elevated levels of this craving lessening hormone, individuals who are stout aren't as delicate with the impacts of leptin and, accordingly, tend not to feel full during and after a dinner. Continuous examination is taking a gander at why leptin messages aren't breaking through to the brain in individuals who are obese.

Weight and insulin

Insulin, a hormone delivered by the pancreas, is significant for the guideline of starches and the digestion of fat. Insulin invigorates glucose (sugar) take-up from the blood in tissues, for example, muscles, the liver and fat. This is a significant procedure to ensure that vitality is accessible for ordinary working and to keep up typical degrees of circling glucose. In an individual who is obese, insulin signals are in some cases lost and tissues are not, at this point ready to control glucose levels. This can prompt the improvement of type II diabetes and metabolic disorder.

Obesity and sex hormones

Muscle versus fat circulation assumes a significant job in the advancement of obesity related conditions, for example, coronary illness, stroke and a few types of joint inflammation. Fat around our mid-region is a higher hazard factor for illness than fat put away on our base, hips and thighs. It appears that oestrogens and androgens help to choose muscle versus fat circulation. Oestrogens are sex hormones made by the ovaries in pre-menopausal ladies. They are answerable for inciting ovulation each menstrual cycle. Men and postmenopausal ladies don't deliver a lot of estrogen in their testicles (balls) or ovaries. Rather, a obese portion of their estrogen is created in their muscle versus fat, in spite of the fact that at much lower sums than what is delivered in pre-menopausal ovaries. In more youthful men, androgens are delivered at significant levels in the testicles. As a man gets more seasoned, these levels steadily decline.

The progressions with age in the sex hormone levels of the two people are related with changes in muscle versus fat dissemination. While ladies of childbearing age will in general store fat in their lower body ('pear-formed'), more seasoned men and postmenopausal ladies will in general increment stockpiling of fat around their mid-region ('apple-molded'). Postmenopausal ladies who are taking estrogen supplements don't collect fat around their mid-region. Creature examines have likewise demonstrated that an absence of estrogen prompts exorbitant weight gain.

Weight and growth hormone

The pituitary organ in our brain produces growth hormone, which impacts an individual's tallness and assists work with boning and muscle. Growth hormone likewise influences digestion (the rate at which we consume kilojoules for vitality). Analysts have discovered that growth hormone levels in individuals who are fat are lower than in individuals of ordinary weight.

Inflammatory factors and obesity

Obesity is additionally connected with second rate ceaseless aggravation inside the fat tissue. Unreasonable fat stockpiling prompts pressure responses inside fat cells, which thus lead to the arrival of master fiery variables from the fat cells themselves and safe cells inside the (fat) tissue.

Obesity hormones as a risk factor for disease

Obesity is related with an expanded danger of various sicknesses, including cardiovascular infection, stroke and a few kinds of malignant growth, and with diminished life span (shorter life expectancy) and lower personal satisfaction. For instance, the expanded creation of oestrogens in the fat of more established ladies who are corpulent is related with an expansion in bosom disease chance, demonstrating that the wellspring of estrogen creation is significant.

Behaviour and obesity hormones

Individuals who are corpulent have hormone levels that support the amassing of muscle to fat ratio. It appears that practices, for example, indulging and absence of standard exercise, after some time, 'reset' the procedures that control craving and muscle versus fat appropriation to make the individual physiologically bound to put on weight. The body is continually trying to look after equalization, so it opposes any transient disturbances, for example, crash abstaining from excessive food intake. Different researchs have demonstrated that an individual's blood leptin level drops after a low-kilojoule diet. Lower leptin levels may build an individual's craving and hinder their digestion. This may assist with clarifying why crash health food nuts as a rule recapture their shed pounds. It is conceivable that leptin treatment may one day help calorie counters to keep up their weight reduction in the long haul, yet more examination is required before this turns into a reality. There is proof to propose that drawn out behaviour changes, for example, good dieting and ordinary exercise, can re-train the body to shed overabundance muscle to fat ratio and keep it off. Studies have likewise indicated that weight reduction because of sound eating regimen and practice or bariatric medical procedure prompts improved insulin opposition, diminished aggravation and gainful balance of obesity hormones. Weight reduction is additionally connected with a diminished danger of creating coronary illness, stroke, type II diabetes and a few tumors.

The Hormone Diet

What is it ?

The hormone diet is a six-week, three-advance procedure intended to adjust hormones and advance a general more advantageous body through eating routine, work out, nourishing enhancements, and detoxification. The eating regimen controls what you eat and furthermore discloses to you the ideal opportunity to eat to guarantee greatest advantage to your hormones.

Stage 1

This piece of the eating regimen includes a fourteen day "detoxification" process. You abstain from eating gluten-containing grains, dairy items produced using bovine's milk, numerous oils, liquor, caffeine, peanuts, sugar, fake sugars, red meat, and citrus natural products. Adequate foods during this stage incorporate normally without gluten grains and starches, most vegetables, most organic products, beans, nuts and seeds, poultry, fish, soy, eggs, plant milks, dairy from sheep or goat, and certain oils. This stage additionally includes taking nourishing enhancements. These incorporate probiotics and mitigating items like turmeric and fish oil.

Stage 2

This stage consolidates a portion of those foods once more into your eating regimen while focusing on how your body reacts to them. In any case, the eating regimen suggests a continuous shirking of "hormone-impeding" foods. These incorporate high fructose corn syrup, fish with high mercury levels, non-natural meats, non-natural espresso, raisins, dates, and peanuts. The full rundown is in the book "The Hormone Diet." The subsequent stage likewise includes freeing your eating regimen of synthetic foods, which include:

- processed foods
- artificial sweeteners
- refined grains
- foods that contain nitrates, such as cured meats, peanut butter, and chocolate

Stage 3

The third stage centers around whole physical and mental wellbeing through cardiovascular exercise and quality preparing. The eating routine arrangement of the subsequent stage proceeds into the third stage.

The Promise

"The Hormone Diet" gloats of being the principal diet book to underscore the significance of hormonal equalization among the entirety of the 16 hormones that impact weight. It additionally claims to be the first to clarify the way of life propensities that can help support hormones to consume fat. These include:

- Sleeping
- eating
- managing Stress
- working out

Counting water weight, the eating regimen focuses on weight reduction of as much as 12 pounds in the principal stage. It focuses on around two pounds every week from that point onward, without calorie checking.

Pros and Cons

The eating routine takes a strong position on weight reduction and in general wellbeing, advancing common, nutritious foods and normal exercise. Likewise, the attention on passionate wellbeing, stress the board, and satisfactory rest are exceptionally significant parts that individuals ought to do, regardless of whether they are on a tight eating routine or not. One significant drawback to the eating routine is its accentuation on a normal measure of weight reduction. An eating regimen plan that suggests 12 pounds of weight reduction in about fourteen days is either ridiculous or impractical. It might likewise prompt weight recapture, in the same way as other different eating regimens.

What You Can Eat

Foods you can eat incorporate lean protein (think chicken bosoms, eggs, and wild-got fish); vegetables and most organic product; chia seeds, flaxseeds, and generally nuts; olive oil and some other unsaturated oils and fats, similar to canola oil; and entire grains like buckwheat, earthy colored rice, and quinoa. On this arrangement, you'll maintain a strategic distance from or limit caffeine, liquor, seared foods, handled meat, peanuts, soaked fat, full-fat dairy, counterfeit sugars, and straightforward high-GI carbs like white bread. You'll eat regularly - each 3-4 hours - settling on solid food decisions in any event 80% of the time. However, you do get one to two "cheat suppers" seven days.

Level of Effort: Medium to High

To start with, you'll quit caffeine, liquor, sugar, dairy, gluten, and most oils for about fourteen days. Additionally, Researchers suggest utilizing pH strips and ketone strips to test your body's pH balance; getting a progression of blood, pee, or spit tests to check hormone levels; and taking enhancements including multivitamins, omega-3 unsaturated fats, and calcium-magnesium-nutrient D3.

Limitations: If you're accustomed to eating arranged suppers and tidbits, The Hormone Diet may be a major change, since it centers around entire foods that you cook yourself. On the off chance that you love espresso or pop, you may think that its difficult to surrender these refreshments for green tea and different beverages on Researchers's rundown.

Cooking and shopping: The arrangement calls for eating natural foods however much as could be expected. The plans and 1-week test menu are genuinely fundamental, so in case you're not happy with cooking the foods in the eating routine arrangement, your choices might be constrained.

Packaged foods or meals: Not required, however Researchers suggest certain brands of enhancements.

In-person meetings: No.

Exercise: Researchers suggest getting approximately 30 minutes of activity 6 days per week in a blend of solidarity preparing, cardio, span preparing, and yoga.

Does It Allow for Dietary Restrictions or Preferences?

Veggie lovers and vegetarians: The eating regimen incorporates protein sources that would work for you.

Gluten-free: You surrender gluten for the initial fourteen days of this eating regimen. From that point forward, gluten isn't totally beyond reach. Researchers encourage perusers to maintain a strategic distance from some handled carbs, similar to white flour and white rice, and to avoid any foods that they believed they had a terrible response to after the detox stage.

Hormone-Diet Strategies

1- Insulin

Insulin is a hormone made in your pancreas, an organ situated behind your stomach. It permits your body to utilize glucose for vitality. Glucose is a kind of sugar found in numerous starches. After a supper or tidbit, the stomach related parcel separates starches and changes them into glucose. Glucose is then consumed into your circulatory system through the covering in your small digestive tract. When glucose is in your circulation system, insulin makes cells all through your body assimilate the sugar and use it for vitality. Insulin additionally helps balance your blood glucose levels. When there's a lot of glucose in your circulation system, insulin flags your body to store the abundance in your liver. The put away glucose isn't discharged until your blood glucose levels decline, for example, between dinners or when your body is focused or needs an additional increase in vitality. Insulin is a hormone delivered by the beta cells of your pancreas. It's emitted in limited quantities for the duration of the day and in bigger sums after suppers. Insulin permits your cells to take in glucose for vitality or capacity, contingent upon what is required at that point. Insulin is additionally the primary fat stockpiling hormone in the body. It advises fat cells to store fat, and keeps put away fat from being separated. At the point when cells are insulin safe (normal), both glucose and insulin levels go up fundamentally. Constantly raised insulin levels (named hyperinsulinemia) can prompt numerous medical issues, including obesity and metabolic disorder. Gorging - particularly sugar, refined starches, and inexpensive food - drives insulin obstruction and expands insulin levels.

Here are a few hints to standardize insulin levels and improve insulin affectability:

- **Stay away from or limit sugar:** High measures of fructose and sucrose advance insulin obstruction and raise insulin levels.
- **Diminish starches:** A low-carb diet can cause a prompt drop in insulin levels.
- **Top off on protein:** Protein really brings insulin up temporarily. In any case, it should prompt long haul decreases in insulin opposition by helping you lose tummy fat.
- **Incorporate a lot of sound fats:** Omega-3 fats found in greasy fish can help lower fasting insulin levels.
- **Exercise routinely:** Overweight ladies who strolled energetically or ran had an improvement

in insulin affectability following 14 weeks in a single report.

- **Get enough magnesium**: Insulin safe individuals are regularly low in magnesium, and magnesium enhancements can improve insulin affectability.
- **Drink green tea:** Green tea may bring down glucose and insulin levels.

10 other Ways to Lower Your Insulin Levels

1. Follow a Low-Carb Diet

Of the three macronutrients — carbs, protein and fat — carbs raise glucose and insulin levels the most. For this and different reasons, low-carb diets can be extremely successful for getting more fit and controlling diabetes. Numerous researchs have affirmed their capacity to bring down insulin levels and increment insulin affectability, contrasted with different weight control plans. Individuals with wellbeing conditions described by insulin opposition, for example, metabolic disorder and polycystic ovary condition (PCOS), may encounter a sensational bringing down of insulin with carb limitation. In one research, people with metabolic disorder were randomized to get either a low-fat or low-carb diet containing 1,500 calories. Insulin levels dropped by a normal of half in the low-carb gathering, contrasted with 19% in the low-fat gathering. In another examination, when ladies with PCOS ate a lower-carb diet containing enough calories to keep up their weight, they encountered more noteworthy decreases in insulin levels than when they ate a higher-carb diet.

2. Take Apple Cider Vinegar

Apple juice vinegar has been credited with forestalling insulin and glucose spikes in the wake of eating. This has been appeared to for the most part happen when vinegar is taken with high-carb foods . A little report found that individuals who took around 2 tablespoons (28 ml) of vinegar with a high-carb dinner experienced lower insulin levels and more prominent sentiments of completion 30 minutes after the supper. Analysts accepted this impact was incompletely because of vinegar's capacity to defer stomach discharging, prompting a progressively slow retention of sugar into the circulation system.

3. Watch Portion Sizes

Despite the fact that the pancreas discharges various measures of insulin relying upon the kind of food you eat, eating a lot of any food at one time can prompt hyperinsulinemia. This is particularly a worry in obese individuals with insulin obstruction. In one research, insulin-safe large individuals who expended a 1,300-calorie supper had double the expansion in insulin as lean individuals who devoured a similar feast. They additionally experienced almost double the expansion in insulin as large individuals who were considered "metabolically solid". Expending less calories has reliably been appeared to build insulin affectability and decline insulin levels in overweight and stout people, paying little mind to the sort of diet they devour. One research took a gander at various weight reduction strategies in 157 individuals with metabolic condition. The scientists found that fasting insulin levels diminished by 16% in the gathering that rehearsed calorie limitation and 12% in the gathering that rehearsed parcel control.

4. Keep away from All Forms of Sugar

Sugar might just be the most significant food to avoid in case you're trying to bring down your insulin levels. In one examination where individuals gorged either treats or peanuts, the sweets bunch encountered a 31% expansion in fasting insulin levels, contrasted with a 12% increment in the nut gathering. In another research, when individuals devoured jams containing high measures of sugar, their insulin levels rose essentially more than in the wake of expending low-sugar jams. Fructose is found in table sugar, nectar, high-fructose corn syrup, agave and syrup. Expending huge amounts of it advances insulin opposition, which at last drives insulin levels higher. One examination found that individuals had comparable insulin reactions in the wake of devouring 50 grams of table sugar, nectar or high-fructose corn syrup consistently for 14 days . In another research, overweight individuals who added high-sugar foods to their standard eating routine encountered a 22% expansion in fasting insulin levels. Conversely, the gathering who added falsely improved foods to their standard eating regimen encountered a 3% decline in fasting insulin levels.

5. Exercise Regularly

Taking part in ordinary physical movement can have ground-breaking insulin-bringing down impacts. Vigorous exercise has all the earmarks of being compelling at expanding insulin affectability in individuals who are corpulent or have type 2 diabetes. One examination analyzed two gatherings. One performed continued vigorous exercise, and the other performed high-power span preparing. The research found that albeit the two gatherings experienced enhancements in wellness, just the gathering that performed continued oxygen consuming action experienced altogether lower insulin levels. There's additionally research demonstrating that obstruction preparing can help decline insulin levels in more established and stationary grown-ups. Consolidating high-impact and opposition practice is by all accounts the best and has been appeared to most extraordinarily influence insulin affectability and levels. In an research of 101 bosom disease survivors, the individuals who occupied with a blend of solidarity preparing and perseverance practice for about four months encountered a 27% decrease in insulin levels.

6. Add Cinnamon to Foods and Beverages

Cinnamon is a delightful flavor stacked with wellbeing advancing cancer prevention agents. Studies in solid individuals and those with insulin obstruction propose that taking cinnamon may improve insulin affectability and abatement insulin levels. In one research, sound individuals who devoured about 1.5 teaspoons of cinnamon in rice pudding had altogether lower insulin reactions than when they ate rice pudding without cinnamon. In another little examination, youngsters who devoured a high-sugar drink in the wake of taking cinnamon for 14 days experienced lower insulin levels than when they expended the beverage subsequent to taking a fake treatment for 14 days. It's essential to take note of that not all researchs have discovered that cinnamon brings down your levels or builds insulin affectability. Cinnamon's belongings may shift from individual to individual. Notwithstanding, including up to one teaspoon (2 grams) every day may give other medical advantages, regardless of whether it doesn't diminish your levels essentially.

7. Avoid Refined Carbs

Refined carbs are a significant piece of numerous individuals' weight control plans. In any case, research in creatures and people has discovered that expending them normally can prompt a few medical issues. These incorporate high insulin levels and weight gain. Moreover, refined carbs have a high glycemic file. The glycemic list (GI) is a scale that quantifies a particular food's ability to raise glucose. Glycemic load considers a food's glycemic record, just as the measure of edible carbs contained in a serving. A few researchs have contrasted foods with various glycemic loads with check whether they influenced insulin levels in an unexpected way. They found that eating a high-glycemic load food raises your levels more than eating a similar bit of a low-glycemic load food, regardless of whether the carb substance of the two foods are comparable. In one research, overweight individuals tailed one of two unlimited calorie eats less for 10 weeks. After a test dinner, the high-GI bunch had higher insulin levels than the low-GI gathering.

8. Avoid Sedentary Behavior

So as to decrease insulin levels, it's essential to carry on with a functioning way of life. One research of more than 1,600 individuals found that the individuals who were the most stationary were about twice as prone to have metabolic disorder as the individuals who performed moderate action in any event 150 minutes of the week. Different examinations have shown that getting up and strolling around, instead of sitting for delayed periods, can help keep insulin levels from spiking after a feast. A 12-week concentrate in moderately aged stationary ladies found that the ladies who strolled for 20 minutes after a huge dinner had expanded insulin affectability, contrasted and ladies who didn't stroll after a feast. Also, the strolling bunch turned out to be increasingly fit and lost muscle versus fat. Another examination took a gander at 113 overweight men in danger of type 2 diabetes. The gathering who made the most strides every day had the best decrease in insulin levels and lost the most gut fat, contrasted with the gathering who made the least number of strides day by day.

9. Try Intermittent Fasting

Discontinuous fasting has gotten well known for weight reduction. Exploration proposes it might help lessen insulin levels as adequately as every day calorie limitation. One research found that corpulent ladies shed pounds and had other wellbeing enhancements following calorie-limited discontinuous fasting with either fluid or strong suppers. Be that as it may, just the fluid eating routine altogether decreased fasting insulin levels. Substitute day fasting includes fasting or drastically lessening calories one day and eating typically the next day. A few researchs have discovered it viably brings down insulin levels. All things considered. Albeit numerous individuals find discontinuous fasting gainful and pleasant, it doesn't work for everybody and may mess up certain individuals.

10.   Increase Soluble Fiber Intake

Dissolvable fiber gives various medical advantages, incorporating assisting with weight reduction and decreasing glucose levels. It assimilates water and structures a gel, which hinders the growth of food through the stomach related plot. This advances sentiments of completion and keeps glucose and insulin from rising excessively fast after a supper. One observational examination discovered ladies who ate the most noteworthy measure of dissolvable fiber were half as prone to be insulin safe as ladies who ate minimal measure of solvent fiber. Solvent fiber additionally helps feed the neighborly microorganisms that live in your colon, which may improve gut wellbeing and diminish insulin obstruction. In a six-week controlled research of stout more seasoned ladies, the individuals who took flaxseed experienced more noteworthy increments in insulin affectability and lower insulin levels than ladies who took a probiotic or fake treatment. By and large, fiber from entire foods seems, by all accounts, to be more powerful at diminishing insulin than fiber in supplement structure, in spite of the fact that outcomes are blended. One research found that a blend of entire food and supplemental fiber brought down insulin levels the most. In the interim, another found that insulin diminished when individuals expended dark beans however not when they took a fiber supplement.

2- Leptin

For patients battling with obesity and weight, hormones regularly influence their general wellbeing. Overabundance muscle versus fat can cause issues with weight and hormonal issues. Leptin is one of the hormones straightforwardly associated with muscle to fat ratio and obesity. Leptin, a hormone discharged from the fat cells situated in fat tissues, imparts signs to the nerve center in the cerebrum. This specific hormone manages and modify long haul food admission and vitality use, not simply starting with one supper then onto the next. The essential plan of leptin is to enable the body to keep up its weight.

Since it originates from fat cells, leptin sums are straightforwardly associated with a person's measure of muscle to fat ratio. In the event that the individual includes muscle versus fat, leptin levels will increment. On the off chance that an individual brings down muscle versus fat ratios, the leptin will diminish too.

What does leptin do?

Leptin is some of the time called the satiety hormone. It represses hunger and control vitality balance, so the body doesn't trigger yearning reactions when it needn't bother with vitality. Nonetheless, when levels of the hormone fall, which happens when an individual gets more fit, the lower levels can trigger gigantic increments in hunger and food desires. This, thus, can make weight reduction increasingly troublesome.

Likely Problems with Leptin

At the point when the body is working appropriately, overabundance fat cells will create leptin, which will trigger the nerve center to bring down the craving, permitting the body to plunge into the fat stores to take care of itself. Tragically, when somebody is stout, that individual will have an excess of leptin in the blood. This can make an absence of affectability the hormone, a condition known as leptin obstruction. Since the individual continues eating, the fat cells produce more leptin to flag the sentiment of satiety, prompting expanded leptin levels.

Low degrees of leptin are uncommon, yet can once in a while happen. For a couple of patients, a condition known as inborn leptin insufficiency shields the body from delivering leptin. Without leptin, the body thinks it has no muscle to fat ratio, and this signs serious, uncontrolled yearning and food consumption. This frequently shows in extreme youth corpulence and deferred adolescence. The treatment for leptin lack is leptin infusions. Leptin is created by your fat cells. It's viewed as a "satiety hormone" that diminishes hunger and causes you to feel full. As a flagging hormone, its job is to speak with the nerve center, the part of your cerebrum that directs hunger and food admission. Leptin tells the cerebrum that there's sufficient fat away and no more is required, which forestalls gorging. Individuals who are overweight or obese for the most part have exceptionally significant levels of leptin in their blood. Truth be told, one examination found that leptin levels in large individuals were multiple times higher than in individuals of ordinary weight. On the off chance that leptin decreases craving, at that point stout individuals with elevated levels of leptin should begin eating less and get more fit. Sadly, in weight the leptin framework doesn't fill in as it should. This is alluded to as leptin obstruction. When leptin flagging is impeded, the message to quit eating doesn't break through to the mind, so it doesn't understand you have enough vitality put away. Fundamentally, your cerebrum thinks it is starving, so you're headed to eat. Leptin levels are likewise decreased when you get more fit, which is one of the principle reasons it is so difficult to keep up weight reduction in the long haul. The mind thinks you are starving, and pushes you to eat more. Two likely reasons for leptin opposition are constantly raised insulin levels and irritation in the nerve center.

Here are a couple of proposals for improving leptin affectability:

- **Keep away from fiery foods**: Limit foods that cause irritation, particularly sweet beverages and trans fats.

- **Eat certain foods**: Eat progressively calming foods, for example, greasy fish.
- Exercise consistently: Moderate action can improve leptin affectability.
- **Get enough rest**: Studies have indicated that deficient rest prompts a drop in leptin levels and expanded hunger.
- **Enhancements**: In one research, ladies on a weight reduction diet who took alpha-lipoic corrosive and fish oil lost more weight and had a littler abatement in leptin than those in a benchmark group.

3- Ghrelin

Weight reduction can be intense, yet keeping up your weight after an eating routine is significantly harder. Exploration shows a huge level of health food nuts recover all the weight they lost inside only one year. Weight re-gain is incompletely because of your body's craving and weight-managing hormones, which try to keep up and even re-increase fat. Ghrelin, the "hunger hormone," assumes a key job since it flags your cerebrum to eat. Its levels increment during an eating regimen and heighten hunger, making it difficult to get in shape.

What is Ghrelin?

Ghrelin is a hormone delivered in the gut. It is frequently named the appetite hormone, and once in a while called lenomorelin. It goes through your circulation system and to your mind, where it advises your cerebrum to get ravenous and search out food. Ghrelin's fundamental capacity is to expand craving. It causes you to expend more food, take in more calories and store fat. What's more, it influences your rest/wake cycle, reward-chasing conduct, taste sensation and starch digestion. This hormone is created in your stomach and discharged when your stomach is unfilled. It enters the circulation system and influences a piece of the cerebrum known as the nerve center, which oversees your hormones and craving. The higher your levels, the hungrier your get. The lower your levels, the more full you feel and the simpler it is to eat less calories.

So in the event that you need to shed pounds, bringing down your ghrelin levels can be valuable. Ghrelin may seem like a horrible, diet-destroying hormone. Be that as it may, in the past it assumed a job in endurance by helping individuals keep up a solid degree of muscle to fat ratio. Nowadays, in the event that you under-eat or battle to put on weight, higher ghrelin levels may assist you with devouring more food and calories every day.

What Causes Ghrelin to Rise?

Ghrelin levels commonly ascend before a dinner, when your stomach is unfilled. At that point they decline not long after, when your stomach is full. While you may expect stout individuals have more elevated levels, they may simply be increasingly delicate to its belongings. Truth be told, some exploration shows their levels are really lower than in lean individuals. Other exploration proposes that corpulent individuals may have an excessively dynamic ghrelin receptor, known as GHS-R, which prompts expanded calorie admission. However paying little heed to how much muscle versus fat you have, ghrelin levels increment and make you hungry when you start an eating routine. This is a characteristic reaction by your body, which trys to shield you from starvation. During an eating routine, your craving increments and your degrees of the "totality hormone" leptin go down. Your metabolic rate likewise will in general diminishing altogether, particularly when you confine calories for significant stretches of time. For evident reasons, these adjustments can make it essentially harder to get thinner and keep it off. Your hormones and digestion change in accordance with try to re-put on all the weight you lost.

How Your Levels Change During a Diet

Inside a day of starting an eating regimen, your ghrelin levels will begin to go up. This change proceeds through the span of weeks. One examination in people found a 24% expansion in ghrelin levels on a 6-month diet. In an additional 3-month weight reduction diet study, analysts found the levels almost multiplied from 770 to 1,322 pmol/liter. During a 6-month lifting weights diet, which achieves an amazingly low degree of muscle to fat ratio through extreme dietary limitations, ghrelin expanded by 40%.

These patterns propose that the more you diet — and the more muscle versus fat and bulk you lose — the higher your levels will rise. This makes you hungrier, so it turns out to be a lot harder to keep up your new weight.

Step by step instructions to Lower Ghrelin and Reduce Hunger

Ghrelin is by all accounts a hormone that can't be legitimately controlled with medications, diets or enhancements. Be that as it may, there are a couple of things you can never really keep up sound levels:

- Dodge weight limits: Both obesity and anorexia modify ghrelin levels.
- Organize rest: Poor rest expands your levels, and has been connected to expanded appetite and weight gain.
- Increment bulk: Higher measures of without fat mass or muscle are related with lower levels.
- Eat more protein: A high-protein diet expands totality and lessens hunger. One of the systems behind this is a decrease in ghrelin levels.
- Keep up a steady weight: Drastic weight changes and yo-yo eating fewer carbs disturb key hormones, including ghrelin.

- Cycle your calories: Periods of more fatty admission can decrease hunger hormones and increment leptin. One examination discovered fourteen days on 29–45% more calories diminished ghrelin levels by 18%.

Ghrelin is known as a "hunger hormone." When your stomach is vacant, it discharges ghrelin, which makes an impression on the nerve center advising you to eat. Regularly, ghrelin levels are most elevated before eating and least about an hour after you've had a dinner. Notwithstanding, in overweight and stout individuals, fasting ghrelin levels are frequently lower than in individuals of typical weight. Studies have likewise indicated that after fat individuals eat a dinner, ghrelin just abatements somewhat. Along these lines, the nerve center doesn't get as solid of a sign to quit eating, which can prompt gorging.

Here are a couple of tips to improve the capacity of ghrelin:

- **Sugar:** Avoid high-fructose corn syrup and sugar-improved beverages, which can impede ghrelin reaction after dinners.

- **Protein:** Eating protein at each dinner, particularly breakfast, can decrease ghrelin levels and advance satiety.

4- Cortisol

Consider cortisol nature's worked in alert framework. It's your body's primary pressure hormone. It works with specific pieces of your mind to control your disposition, inspiration, and dread. Your adrenal organs - triangle-formed organs at the head of your kidneys - make cortisol. It's most popular for helping fuel your body's "battle or-flight" intuition in an emergency, yet cortisol assumes a significant job in various things your body does. For instance, it:

- Oversees how your body utilizes starches, fats, and proteins
- Holds aggravation down
- Directs your circulatory strain
- Builds your (glucose)
- Controls your rest/wake cycle

- Lifts vitality so you can deal with pressure and reestablishes harmony a short time later

How Can It Work?

Your nerve center and pituitary organ - both situated in your mind - can detect if your blood contains the correct degree of cortisol. On the off chance that the level is excessively low, your mind modifies the measure of hormones it makes. Your adrenal organs get on these signs. At that point, they calibrate the measure of cortisol they discharge. Cortisol receptors - which are in many cells in your body - get and utilize the hormone in various manners. Your requirements will vary from everyday. For example, when your body is on high ready, cortisol can adjust or close down capacities that disrupt everything. These might incorporate your stomach related or conceptive frameworks, your invulnerable framework, or even your growth forms. Now and again, your cortisol levels can escape whack.

A lot of Stress

After the weight or peril has passed, your cortisol level should quiet down. Your heart, circulatory strain, and other body frameworks will return to typical.

However, consider the possibility that you're under consistent pressure and the caution button remains on.

It can wreck your body's most significant capacities. It can likewise prompt various medical issues, including:

- Nervousness and misery
- Migraines
- Coronary illness

- Memory and fixation issues

- Issues with assimilation

- Inconvenience resting

- Weight gain

- An excessive amount of Cortisol

A knob (mass) in your adrenal organ or a tumor in the mind's pituitary organ can trigger your body to make a lot of cortisol. This can cause a condition called Cushing disorder. It can prompt fast weight gain, skin that wounds effectively, muscle shortcoming, diabetes, and numerous other medical issues.

Too Little Cortisol

On the off chance that your body doesn't make enough of this hormone, you have a condition specialists call Addison's illness. As a rule, the indications show up after some time. They include:

- Changes in your skin, such as obscuring on scars and in skin folds
- Being worn out constantly
- Muscle shortcoming that deteriorates
- Looseness of the bowels, queasiness, and retching
- Loss of craving and weight
- Low circulatory strain

Cortisol is a hormone delivered by the adrenal organs. It's known as a "stress hormone" since it's discharged when your body detects pressure. Like different hormones, it's essential to endurance. In any case, incessantly raised degrees of cortisol can prompt gorging and weight gain. Apparently ladies who heft overabundance weight around the center react to worry with a more prominent increment in cortisol. Be that as it may, a severe eating regimen can likewise raise cortisol. In one research, ladies who expended a low-calorie diet had higher cortisol levels and announced inclination more worried than ladies who ate a typical eating routine.

These techniques can lessen cortisol levels:

Adjusted eating regimen: Follow a fair, genuine food-based eating routine. Try not to slice calories to very low levels.

Meditate: Practicing contemplation can essentially diminish cortisol creation .

Tune in to music: Specialists report that while calming music is played during clinical methods, cortisol doesn't ascend so a lot.

Rest progressively: One research found that when pilots lost 15 hours of rest through the span of seven days, their cortisol levels expanded by 50-80%

5- Estrogen

Estrogen is a hormone that assumes different jobs in the body. In females, it creates and keep up both the conceptive framework and female qualities, for example, bosoms and pubic hair. Estrogen adds to intellectual wellbeing, bone wellbeing, the capacity of the cardiovascular framework, and other basic substantial procedures. Notwithstanding, the vast majority know it for its job nearby progesterone in female sexual and regenerative wellbeing. The ovaries, adrenal organs, and fat tissues produce estrogen. Both female and male bodies have this hormone, yet females make a greater amount of it.

Sorts of estrogen

There are various sorts of estrogen:

Estrone

This sort of estrogen is available in the body after menopause. It is a more fragile type of estrogen and one that the body can change over to different types of estrogen, as essential.

Estradiol

The two guys and females produce estradiol, and it is the most widely recognized sort of estrogen in females during their regenerative years. A lot of estradiol may bring about skin break out, loss of sex drive, osteoporosis, and discouragement. High levels can build the danger of uterine and bosom malignancy. Be that as it may, low levels can bring about weight gain and cardiovascular illness.

Estriol

Levels of estriol ascend during pregnancy, as it enables the uterus to develop and readies the body for conveyance. Estriol levels top not long before birth.

Function

Estrogen empowers the accompanying organs to work:

Ovaries: Estrogen animates the growth of the egg follicle.

Vagina: In the vagina, estrogen keeps up the thickness of the vaginal divider and advances oil.

Uterus: Estrogen upgrades and keeps up the mucous film that lines the uterus. It additionally directs the stream and thickness of uterine bodily fluid emissions.

Bosoms: The body utilizes estrogen in the arrangement of bosom tissue. This hormone likewise helps stop the progression of milk in the wake of weaning.

Levels of estrogen

Estrogen levels shift among people. They additionally vary during the menstrual cycle and over a female's lifetime. This variance can at times produce impacts, for example, mind-set changes before feminine cycle or hot blazes in menopause.

Factors that can influence estrogen levels include:

- pregnancy, the finish of pregnancy, and breastfeeding
- adolescence
- menopause
- more established age
- overweight and obesity

- extraordinary abstaining from excessive food intake or anorexia nervosa
- arduous exercise or preparing
- the utilization of specific meds, including steroids, ampicillin, estrogen-containing medications, phenothiazines, and antibiotic medications
- some innate conditions, for example, Turner's disorder
- hypertension
- diabetes
- essential ovarian inadequacy
- an underactive pituitary organ
- polycystic ovary condition (PCOS)
- tumors of the ovaries or adrenal organs

Estrogen impalance

An impalance of estrogen prompts:

- unpredictable or no monthly cycle
- light or overwhelming seeping during monthly cycle
- progressively serious premenstrual or menopausal side effects

- hot glimmers, night sweats, or both
- noncancerous bumps in the bosom and uterus
- state of mind changes and resting issues
- weight gain, basically in the hips, thighs, and midsection
- low sexual want
- vaginal dryness and vaginal decay
- weakness
- disposition swings
- sentiments of melancholy and nervousness
- dry skin
- A portion of these impacts are basic during menopause.

Some innate and different conditions can prompt significant levels of estrogen in guys, which can result in:

- finfertility
- erectile brokenness
- bigger bosoms, known as gynecomastia

Guys with low estrogen levels may have abundance midsection fat and low charisma.

Estrogen is the most significant female sex hormone. It is for the most part delivered by the ovaries, and is associated with managing the female regenerative framework. Both extremely high and low degrees of estrogen can prompt weight gain. This relies upon age, activity of different hormones, and generally condition of wellbeing. To keep up ripeness during the conceptive years, estrogen begins advancing fat stockpiling at pubescence. Also, it might invigorate fat addition in the primary portion of pregnancy . Obese ladies will in general have higher estrogen levels than ordinary weight ladies, and a few specialists accept this is because of natural impacts. During menopause, when estrogen levels drop in light of the fact that less is created in the ovaries, the site for fat stockpiling shifts from the hips and thighs to instinctive fat in the midsection. This advances insulin obstruction and expands illness chance .

These foods and way of life techniques can help oversee estrogen:

Fiber: Eat a lot of fiber on the off chance that you need to decrease estrogen levels.

Cruciferous vegetables: Eating cruciferous vegetables may effectsly affect estrogen.

Flax seeds: Although the phytoestrogens in them are disputable, flax seeds seem to effectsly affect estrogen in most ladies.

Exercise: Physical movement can help standardize estrogen levels in both premenopausal and postmenopausal ladies.

6- Neuropeptide Y (NPY)

Neuropeptide Y (NPY) is a polypeptide containing 36 amino acids. Circling NPY begins transcendently from the sympatho-adrenomedullary sensory system. It has a vasoconstrictive and mitogenic impact on veins and is by all accounts engaged with circulatory strain guideline and angiogenesis. NPY is a strong orexigenic specialist and is tryed to assume a main job in the guideline of eating conduct. Incitement of the NPY-ergic arcuate – paraventricular core (ARC–PVN) pathway by work out, fasting, vitality misfortune (glucosuria) is trailed by expanded hunger and food consumption and expanded parasympathetic movement, yet concealment of thoughtful action and vitality use. The final product of this procedure is an expansion of vitality stores. Action of the NPY-ergic ARC–PVN pathway is stifled by leptin – a polypeptide delivered by adipocytes. Albeit working of a NPY-leptin criticism was found in rodents, it appears to be likely that likewise in man the NPY–leptin hub is engaged with the guideline of food admission and vitality use.

Neuropeptide Y (NPY) is a hormone created by cells in the mind and sensory system. It invigorates hunger, especially for sugars, and is most elevated during times of fasting or food hardship. Levels of neuropeptide Y are raised during times of pressure, which can prompt gorging and stomach fat addition .

Recommendations for lowering NPY:

Eat enough protein: Eating too little protein has been appeared to expand arrival of NPY, which prompts hunger, expanded food admission and weight gain.

Don't fast for too long: Animal examinations have shown that extremely long diets, for example, more than 24 hours, can drastically expand NPY levels.

Soluble fiber: Eating a lot of solvent prebiotic fiber to take care of the cordial microscopic organisms in the gut may lessen NPY levels.

7- Growth hormone

Growth hormone (GH), additionally called somatotropin or human growth hormone, peptide hormone emitted by the foremost flap of the pituitary organ. It animates the growth of basically all tissues of the body, including bone. GH is blended and emitted by front pituitary cells called somatotrophs, which discharge somewhere in the range of one and two milligrams of the hormone every day. GH is essential for typical physical growth in kids; its levels rise logically during adolescence and top during the growth spray that happens in pubescence.

In biochemical terms, GH invigorates protein blend and expands fat breakdown to give the vitality important to tissue growth. It likewise threatens (restricts) the activity of insulin. GH may act straightforwardly on tissues, yet quite a bit of its impact is interceded by incitement of the liver and different tissues to deliver and discharge insulin-like growth factors, fundamentally insulin-like growth factor 1 (IGF-1; previously called somatomedin). The term insulin-like growth factor is gotten from the capacity of high groupings of these elements to mirror the activity of insulin, in spite of the fact that their essential activity is to animate growth. Serum IGF-1 fixations increment dynamically with age in youngsters, with a quickened increment at the hour of the pubertal growth spray. After pubescence the groupings of IGF-1 bit by bit decline with age, as do GH focuses. GH discharge is invigorated by growth hormone-discharging hormone (GHRH) and is hindered by somatostatin. Moreover, GH discharge is pulsatile, with floods in emission happening after the beginning of profound rest that are particularly noticeable at the hour of pubescence. In typical subjects, GH discharge increments in light of diminished food admission and to physiological burdens and diminishes because of food ingestion. Be that as it may, a few people are influenced by variations from the norm in GH emission, which include either insufficiency or excess of the hormone.

10 Strategies to Boost Human Growth Hormone (HGH) Naturally.

1- Lose body fat

The measure of stomach fat you convey is straightforwardly identified with your HGH creation .Those with more significant levels of midsection fat will probably have impeded HGH creation and an expanded danger of sickness.One research saw that those with multiple times the measure of midsection fat as the benchmark group had not exactly a large portion of their measure of HGH .Another research observed the 24-hour arrival of HGH and found an enormous decrease in those with increasingly stomach fat. Strikingly, research proposes that abundance muscle to fat ratio influences HGH levels more in men. In any case, bringing down muscle to fat ratio is as yet key for the two sexual orientations. Likewise, an examination found that individuals with heftiness had lower levels of HGH and IGF-1 — a development related protein. In the wake of losing a lot of weight, their levels came back to typical.

Stomach fat is the most hazardous sort of put away fat and connected to numerous ailments. Losing midsection fat will help upgrade your HGH levels and different parts of your wellbeing.

2- Fast intermittently

Studies show that fasting prompts a significant increment in HGH levels.One research found that 3 days into a quick, HGH levels expanded by over 300%. Following multi week of fasting, they had expanded by a huge 1,250%. Different examinations have discovered comparative impacts, with twofold or triple HGH levels after only 2–3 days of fasting .In any case, constant fasting isn't maintainable in the long haul. Irregular fasting is a progressively well known dietary methodology that limits eating to short timespans.Numerous strategies for discontinuous fasting are accessible. One basic methodology is a day by day 8-hour eating window with a 16-hour quick. Another includes eating just 500–600 calories 2 days out of each week. Irregular fasting can help improve HGH levels in two fundamental manners. To start with, it can assist you with dropping muscle versus fat, which legitimately influences HGH creation. Second, it'll keep your insulin levels low for the greater part of the day, as insulin is discharged when you eat. Exploration proposes that insulin spikes can upset your regular development hormone creation.One research watched huge contrasts in HGH levels on the fasting day contrasted and the eating day. Shorter 12–

16-hour diets likely assistance too, however more examination is expected to contrast their belongings and entire day diets.

3- Try an arginine supplement

At the point when taken alone, arginine may help HGH. In spite of the fact that the vast majority will in general utilize amino acids like arginine close by work out, a few examinations show next to zero increment in HGH levels. Nonetheless, contemplates have seen that taking arginine all alone — with no activity — fundamentally builds levels of this hormone . Other non-practice concentrates additionally bolster the utilization of arginine to help HGH. One research analyzed the impacts of taking either 45 or 114 mg of arginine for every pound (100 or 250 mg for each kg) of body weight, or around 6–10 or 15–20 grams for every day, individually. It found no impact for the lower portion, yet members taking the higher portion experienced around a 60% expansion in HGH levels during rest.

4. Decrease your sugar intake

An expansion in insulin is related with lower HGH levels. Refined carbs and sugar raise insulin levels the most, so decreasing your admission may help enhance development hormone levels. One research found that sound individuals had 3–4 times higher HGH levels than those with diabetes, just as hindered carb resilience and insulin work. Alongside legitimately influencing insulin levels, abundance sugar admission is a key factor in weight addition and stoutness, which additionally influence HGH levels.All things considered, the intermittent sweet treat won't sway your HGH levels in the long haul.Plan to accomplish a reasonable eating regimen, as what you eat profoundly affects your wellbeing, hormones, and body creation.

5. Try not to eat alot before sleep time

Your body normally discharges noteworthy measures of HGH, particularly around evening time.Given that most dinners cause an ascent in insulin levels, a few specialists propose staying away from food before sleep time. Specifically, a high-carb or high-protein dinner may spike your insulin and conceivably hinder a portion of the HGH discharged around evening time. Remember that deficient exploration exists on this hypothesis. By the by, insulin levels typically decline 2–3 hours subsequent to eating, so you may wish to maintain a strategic distance from carb-or protein-based suppers 2–3 hours before sleep time.

6. Take a GABA supplement

Gamma aminobutyric corrosive (GABA) is a non-protein amino corrosive that capacities as a synapse, imparting signs around your cerebrum.As a notable quieting specialist for your mind and focal sensory system, it's regularly used to help rest. Strangely, it might likewise help increment your HGH levels.One research found that taking a GABA supplement prompted a 400% expansion in HGH very still and a 200% increment following activity.GABA may likewise build HGH levels by improving your rest, since your evening time development hormone discharge is connected to rest quality and profundity.Be that as it may, the majority of these increments were fleeting and GABA's drawn out advantages for development hormone levels stay muddled.

7. Exercise at a high intensity

Exercise is one of the best approaches to fundamentally raise your HGH levels.The expansion relies upon the kind of activity, force, food consumption around the exercise, and your body's own characteristics.High-force practice expands HGH the most, however all types of activity are gainful.You can perform rehashed runs, span preparing, weight preparing, or high-intensity aerobics to spike your HGH levels and expand fat misfortune. Likewise with supplements, practice essentially causes momentary spikes in HGH levels. All things considered, over the long haul, exercise may enhance your hormone capacity and abatement muscle versus fat, the two of which will profit your HGH levels.

8. Take beta-alanine and/or a sports drink around your workouts

A few games enhancements can improve execution and briefly help your HGH levels.In one examination, taking 4.8 grams of beta-alanine before an exercise expanded the quantity of reiterations performed by 22%.It additionally multiplied pinnacle power and supported HGH levels contrasted and the non-supplement gathering. Another examination exhibited that a sweet games drink expanded HGH levels close to the furthest limit of an exercise. Be that as it may, in case you're trying to lose fat, the beverage's additional calories will refute any profit by the present moment HGH spike. Studies have demonstrated that protein shakes — both with and without carbs — can help HGH levels around exercises. Notwithstanding, if a casein or whey protein supplement is taken preceding quality exercise, it might have the contrary impact.

9. Optimize your Sleep

Most of HGH is discharged in beats when you rest. These heartbeats depend on your body's inside clock or circadian musicality.The biggest heartbeats happen before 12 PM, with some littler heartbeats in the early morning.Studies have demonstrated that helpless rest can lessen the measure of HGH your body produces. Indeed, getting a satisfactory measure of profound rest is perhaps the best technique to improve your long haul HGH creation. Here are a couple of straightforward techniques to help upgrade your rest:

- Stay away from blue light presentation before sleep time.
- Peruse a book at night.
- Ensure your room is at an agreeable temperature.
- Try not to devour caffeine late in the day.

10. Take a melatonin supplement

Melatonin is a hormone that assumes a significant job in rest and circulatory strain guideline. Melatonin supplements have become a well known tranquilizer that can build the quality and span of your rest. While great rest alone may profit HGH levels, further examination has indicated that a melatonin supplement can legitimately improve HGH creation. Melatonin is likewise genuinely protected and non-poisonous. Be that as it may, it might modify your cerebrum science here and there, so you might need to check with your social insurance supplier before utilizing it. To amplify its belongings, take 1–5 mg around 30 minutes before bed. Start with a lower portion to survey your resilience, at that point increment if necessary.

8- Thyroid

For overweight and fat patients, incorporating those with type 2 diabetes, clinicians presently have a viable strategy for surveying which patients may be urged to consider dietary acclimations to turn around their overabundance body weight, while others may have more affirmation that bariatric medical procedure offers a superior long haul viewpoint for weight loss. Results from this randomized clinical preliminary give a solid sign that even in grown-ups with typical thyroid capacity, these hormones assume a job in body weight guideline and may help recognize people progressively receptive to a dietary mediation planned for elevating weight loss, as indicated by lead examiner Qi Sun, MD, ScD, an associate educator of sustenance at the Harvard University School of Public Health in Boston, Massachusetts. Scientists found that higher pattern free triiodothyronine (T3) and free thyroxine (T4) levels anticipated more weight reduction among overweight and corpulent grown-ups with typical thyroid capacity. Lamentably, these hormones couldn't offer any hint with regards to whether these people would recapture the shed pounds, said Dr. Sun.

Linking Thyroid Hormones and Body Weight

"Our examination was among the first to explore the job of thyroid hormones in weight change in a controlled clinical preliminary instead of an observational investigation," Dr. Sun, MD, ScD, told EndocrineWeb. More significant levels of gauge free T3 and free T4, yet not TSH, had an essentially related to more prominent weight reduction at six and two years, actuated by weight reduction dietary plans. Notwithstanding, pattern TSH didn't foresee weight reduction or weight recover. Furthermore, changes in free T3 and all out T3 levels, yet not free T4 and all out

T4 or TSH, were decidedly connected with changes in body weight and metabolic boundaries, including RMR, circulatory strain, triglycerides, and leptin. "Realizing which components can anticipate weight reduction expands our comprehension of the science of [body weight regulation], just as to recognize high-hazard patients right off the bat who may need to think about different alternatives, for example, bariatric medical procedure," Dr. Sun told EndocrineWeb. "This is a significant investigation," said J. Michael Gonzalez-Campoy, MD, PhD, clinical chief and Chief Executive Officer of the Minnesota Center for Obesity, Metabolism and Endocrinology in Eagan, Minnesota, told EndocrineWeb, "It approves that there is a job for thyroid hormones in tending to weight reduction and weight support." Members in an additional 2-year randomized clinical trial were evaluated for changes in body weight and resting metabolic rate (RMR) during the intercession time frame, which offered results information for the POUNDS LOST convention. In this examination, freeT3, free T4, absolute T3, all out T4, and thyroid-animating hormone (TSH), just as anthropometric estimations and biochemical boundaries were evaluated at pattern, a half year, and 24 months. The mean age of the 569 members was 51.6 (± 9.0) years, and their mean BMI was 32.6 (± 3.8). They lost a normal of 6.6 kg during the initial a half year, and in this way recovered a normal of 2.7 kg for the staying 6 two year time frame. There were no huge contrasts in weight reduction among the four distinct eating regimens concentrated in the POUNDS LOST trial. In this analysis, study members gave fasting serum tests at gauge and a half year, and 429 of those members likewise gave blood tests at two years.

5 Foods That Improve Thyroid Function

While the reason for thyroid issues is to a great extent obscure, there is proof that specific foods can help in thyroid capacity. In the event that you have hypothyroidism, here are five foods to add to your eating regimen.

Roasted seaweed

seaweed growth, for example, kelp, nori, and wakame, are normally wealthy in iodine—a minor component required for typical thyroid capacity. Eat seaweed growth with sushi or get bundled kelp bites to prepare in plates of mixed greens.

Salted nuts

Brazil nuts, macadamia nuts, and hazelnuts are superb wellsprings of selenium, which helps bolster solid thyroid capacity. Gather a little sack of arranged nuts to nibble on for the duration of the day.

Baked fish

Fish is wealthy in Omega-3 unsaturated fats and selenium, which both assistance decline irritation. Prepare salmon, cod, ocean bass, haddock, or roost for lunch or supper to get a sound portion of Omega-3s and selenium.

Frozen yogurt

Dairy items like yogurt, frozen yogurt, and milk contain iodine. The thyroid needs iodine to keep its organs from getting amplified—known as goiter. Treat yourself to a low-fat serving of solidified yogurt to get adequate degrees of iodine.

Fresh eggs

Eggs contain solid measures of both selenium and iodine. For the most medical advantages, eat the entire egg, as the yolk holds the greater part of the supplements.

9- **Testosterone**

What Is Testosterone?

Testosterone is the most significant male sex hormone. It is chiefly created by the gonads in men and ovaries in ladies. Hormones are errand person atoms that assume an essential job in all body frameworks. They are discharged into the circulatory system, which conveys them to their objective cells. At the point when hormones interact with good cells, they tie to receptors on their surface and influence their capacity. Testosterone's fundamental job is to advance male qualities like a more profound voice, expanded bulk, more grounded bones and facial and body hair development.

Satisfactory levels are likewise fundamental for the development of sperm cells and the support of male fruitfulness. Obviously, testosterone levels are a lot higher in men than in ladies. However the hormone assumes a few imperative jobs in ladies, as well. One of its most significant capacities in the two sexual orientations is to keep up bulk and advance muscle development and bone quality. Your levels decrease with age, somewhat clarifying age-related muscle and bone misfortune. In addition to the fact that deficiency suppresses muscle development and upkeep, however it might likewise advance weight gain.

Insufficiency May Lead to Weight Gain

Testosterone advances muscle development. Simultaneously, it might smother fat addition . Accordingly, some testosterone-inadequate men will in general increase fat more effectively than their sound friends . Muscles consume unmistakably a larger number of calories than fat tissue. Absence of muscle hence puts individuals at a higher danger of eating excessively and putting away the overabundance calories as fat. Indeed, a few specialists accept that diminished bulk is the essential explanation lack prompts weight gain in men.

Weight Is Linked With Low Levels

By and large, corpulent men have 30% lower testosterone levels than the individuals who are typical weight. Over 70% of excessively fat men experience the ill effects of male hypogonadism, or testosterone insufficiency, a confusion portrayed by unusually low degrees of this hormone. Male hypogonadism may turn around with weight reduction. Researchers are not so much sure why levels are lower in corpulent men, however most examinations highlight the accompanying procedures. To begin with, tummy fat contains significant levels of the protein aromatase, which changes over testosterone into estrogen, the female sex hormone. This clarifies why hefty men have higher estrogen levels than ordinary weight men. Second, high aromatase and estrogen action lessens the creation of gonadotropin-discharging hormone (GRH). Absence of GRH prompts lower levels of luteinizing hormone, which thus diminishes the creation of testosterone. Set forth plainly, exorbitant stomach fat seems to smother testosterone levels.

Do Supplements Cause Weight Loss?

The expression "testosterone supplement" can allude to three things: unlawful anabolic steroids, testosterone substitution treatment and testosterone supporters.

Illegal Anabolic Steroids

Engineered steroids identified with testosterone are all things considered known as anabolic steroids. The term may likewise allude to testosterone itself. A few weight lifters abuse anabolic steroids to build testosterone past typical levels and lift muscle development. However manhandling anabolic steroids is unlawful in numerous nations, including the US. Solid men with ordinary testosterone levels ought not take anabolic steroids in any structure, since long haul abuse can cause antagonistic reactions. These incorporate sexual brokenness, forceful conduct, liver issues and coronary illness. A few analysts have called attention to that not these reactions apply to testosterone itself but instead to its manufactured subsidiaries. Actually, testosterone assumes a substantial job in the treatment of some ailments. For example, it is legitimately recommended to standardize testosterone levels in inadequate men, a treatment known as testosterone substitution treatment. While substantial testosterone substitution treatment may advance weight reduction in stout men, anabolic steroid abuse isn't a suggested weight reduction methodology. Extreme bulk might be hard to keep up in the long haul and unused muscles will in general transform into fat after some time.

Testosterone Replacement Therapy

This hormone is regularly lawfully endorsed to treat testosterone inadequacy (hypogonadism) or other ailments.

The treatment is known as testosterone substitution treatment and is performed under clinical watch. It very well may be controlled as an enhancement, skin fix, cream or infusion. There is some proof that substitution treatment can prompt weight reduction in hefty patients with testosterone lack. One 56-week concentrate in 100 large men on a diminished calorie diet found that infusions improved weight reduction by 6.4 pounds (2.9 kg) contrasted with the individuals who didn't get any treatment. While the two gatherings lost bulk just as fat mass on a low-calorie diet, testosterone caused critical muscle recapture during the weight support period.

It prompts weight reduction by advancing muscle development, which thus builds the quantity of calories consumed. It might likewise lessen weakness, upgrade inspiration and advance more prominent physical action. These elements assume a significant job in weight reduction. Remember that these examinations analyzed the impacts of substitution treatment in lacking men under clinical watch. There is no proof that substitution treatment causes weight reduction in solid men with ordinary testosterone levels.

Testosterone Boosters

Otherwise called "common testosterone supplements," testosterone promoters increment the regular creation of this hormone inside your body. These enhancements don't contain any testosterone and are typically plant-based. A few promoters, for example, ashwagandha, D-aspartic corrosive and fenugreek seed remove, may raise testosterone levels and improve muscle development in men who have low levels, in spite of the fact that the proof is conflicting. Be that as it may, a significant number of the wellbeing claims related with promoters are not upheld by science. For example, Tribulus terrestris, an enhancement generally sold as a sponsor, doesn't seem to raise levels.

Presently, no examinations have demonstrated huge weight reduction with testosterone sponsors, albeit some will in general decrease fat mass.

How Might You Increase Your Levels Naturally?

The fundamental indications of testosterone inadequacy incorporate low drive, trouble keeping up or building up an erection and less serious climaxes. Different manifestations incorporate exhaustion, low mind-set and diminished bulk. On the off chance that you speculate you have low levels, a basic blood test can affirm insufficiency. Substitution treatment is the best treatment. Be that as it may, it is dubious and has hazards just as advantages.

Luckily, there are a few different ways you can normally improve low testosterone levels.

A couple of strategies are recorded beneath:

- **Strength train:** Many examinations show that quality preparing can build your degrees of this hormone.
- **Take Vitamin D supplements:** Vitamin D lack is related with low levels. Enhancements can take levels back to ordinary.
- **Get adequate zinc:** Deficiency in zinc may lessen levels. Eat a lot of zinc-rich foods, for example, meat, nuts and seeds, to standardize your levels.
- **Get enough Sleep:** Poor rest is related with a drop in levels. Truth be told, getting enough rest is one of the most significant parts of a sound way of life.
- **Try ashwagandha:** The restorative spice ashwagandha, referred to deductively as Withania somnifera, may improve levels and richness.
- **Relax and minimize stress:** Chronic pressure raises the degrees of cortisol, a hormone that may

smother testosterone levels. A tranquil domain and loosening up interest exercises are a foundation of a sound way of life.

Notwithstanding raising your testosterone levels, the above methodologies can improve your overall wellbeing. Some may even assist you with shedding pounds, particularly when joined with other weight reduction techniques.

10 Strategies to Boost Your Metabolism

Boosting digestion is the sacred goal of weight watchers all over, however how quick your body consumes calories relies upon a few things. A few people acquire a rapid digestion. Men will in general consume a larger number of calories than ladies, even while resting. What's more, for a great many people, digestion eases back consistently after age 40. In spite of the fact that you can't control your age, sex, or hereditary qualities, there are different approaches to improve your digestion. Here are 10 of them.

Build Muscle

Your body continually consumes calories, in any event, when you're sitting idle. This resting metabolic rate is a lot higher in individuals with more muscle. Each pound of muscle utilizes around 6 calories every day just to continue itself, while each pound of fat consumes just 2 calories day by day. That little distinction can include after some time. After a meeting of solidarity preparing, muscles are actuated all over your body, raising your normal day by day metabolic rate.

Step Up Your Workout

High-impact exercise may not fabricate huge muscles, yet it can fire up your digestion in the hours after an exercise. The key is to propel yourself. High-force practice conveys a greater, longer ascent in resting metabolic rate than low-or moderate-power exercises. To get the advantages, try a progressively extraordinary class at the rec center or incorporate short eruptions of running during your standard walk.

Fuel Up With Water

Your body needs water to process calories. On the off chance that you are even somewhat dried out, your digestion may back off. In one investigation, grown-ups who drank at least eight glasses of water a day consumed a greater number of calories than the individuals who drank four. To remain hydrated, drink a glass of water or other unsweetened refreshment before each supper and tidbit. Additionally, nibble on new leafy foods, which normally contain water, as opposed to pretzels or chips.

Try Energy Drinks

A few fixings in caffeinated beverages can give your digestion a lift. They're brimming with caffeine, which expands the measure of vitality your body employments. They now and then have taurine, an amino corrosive. Taurine can accelerate your digestion and may help consume fat. In any case, utilizing these beverages can cause issues like hypertension, nervousness, and rest issues for certain individuals. The American Academy of Pediatrics doesn't suggest them for children and youngsters.

Snack Smart

Eating all the more frequently can assist you with getting in shape. At the point when you eat enormous suppers with numerous hours in the middle of, your digestion eases back down between dinners. Having a little feast or nibble each 3 to 4 hours keeps your digestion turning, so you consume more calories through the span of a day. A few examinations have likewise demonstrated that individuals who nibble normally eat less at supper time.

Spice Up Your Meals

Fiery foods have common synthetic concoctions that can kick your digestion into a higher apparatus. Cooking foods with a tablespoon of hacked red or green bean stew pepper can support your metabolic rate. The impact is likely transitory, yet in the event that you eat hot foods regularly, the advantages may include. For a brisk lift, flavor up pasta dishes, bean stew, and stews with red pepper chips.

Power up with Protein

Your body consumes a lot a bigger number of calories processing protein than it does eating fat or sugars. As a feature of a decent eating routine, supplanting some carbs with lean, protein-rich foods can support digestion at supper time. Great wellsprings of protein incorporate lean hamburger, turkey, fish, white meat chicken, tofu, nuts, beans, eggs, and low-fat dairy items.

Sip Some Black Coffee

In case you're an espresso consumer, you most likely appreciate the vitality and focus advantages. Taken with some restraint, one of espresso's advantages might be a momentary ascent in your metabolic rate. Caffeine can assist you with feeling less drained and even increment your continuance while you work out.

Energize With Green Tea

Drinking green tea or oolong tea offers the joined advantages of caffeine and catechins, substances appeared to fire up the digestion for two or three hours. Examination proposes that drinking 2 to 4 cups of either tea may push the body to consume 17% more calories during respectably extreme exercise for a brief timeframe.

Avoid Crash Diets

Crash abstains from food - those including eating less than 1,200 (in case you're a lady) or 1,800 (in case you're a man) calories daily - are awful for anybody planning to enliven their digestion. In spite of the fact that these weight control plans may assist you with dropping pounds, that comes to the detriment of good food. Furthermore, it reverse discharges, since you can lose muscle, which thusly eases back your digestion.

The conclusive outcome is your body consumes less calories and puts on weight quicker than before the eating regimen.

10 Tips to Best Hormone Diet ever

1: Drink a lot of water or other without calorie refreshments

Before you attack that sack of potato chips, drink a glass of water first. Individuals in some cases mistake hunger for hunger, so you can wind up eating additional calories when a super cold glass of water is actually all you required. In the event that plain water doesn't cut it, have a go at drinking seasoned shining water or preparing some natural product mixed home grown tea.

2: Be selective about evening snacks

Thoughtless eating happens most every now and again after supper, when you at long last plunk down and unwind. Eating before the TV is probably the least demanding approaches to lose your eating regimen course. Either close down the kitchen following a specific hour, or permit yourself a low-calorie nibble, similar to a 100-calorie pack of treats or a half-cup scoop of low-fat frozen yogurt.

3: Enjoy your preferred food

Rather than removing your preferred food inside and out, be a thin customer. Get one new pastry kitchen treat rather than a case, or a little segment of sweets from the mass containers rather than an entire pack. You can in any case make the most of your preferred food - the key is control.

4: Eat a few smaller than usual suppers during the day

In the event that you eat less calories than you consume, you'll get in shape. Be that as it may, when you're eager constantly, eating less calories can be a test. "Studies show individuals who eat 4-5 suppers or snacks for each day are better ready to control their craving and weight," says stoutness specialist Rebecca Reeves, DrPH, RD. She suggests separating your every day calories into littler suppers or snacks and getting a charge out of the greater part of them prior in the day - supper ought to be the last time you eat.

5: Eat protein at each feast

Protein is a definitive top me-off food - it's more fulfilling than carbs or fats and keeps you feeling full for more. It additionally assists save with muscling mass and empowers fat consuming. So make certain to fuse solid proteins like fish, lean meat, egg whites, yogurt, cheddar, soy, nuts, or beans into your dinners and bites.

6: Stock your kitchen with solid, helpful food

Having prepared to-eat tidbits and suppers in-minutes available sets you up for progress. You'll be less inclined to hit the drive-through or request a pizza on the off chance that you can put together a sound feast in five or 10 minutes. Here are a few fundamentals to keep close by: solidified vegetables, entire grain pasta, diminished fat cheddar, canned tomatoes, canned beans, pre-cooked flame broiled chicken bosom, entire grain tortillas or pitas, and sacks of plate of mixed greens.

7: Order kids' bits at eateries

Requesting a kid size dish is an incredible method to cut calories and keep your segments sensible. This has become such a well known pattern, that most servers won't hesitate when you request off the children's menu. Another stunt is to utilize littler plates. This enables the parts to look like more, and if your brain is fulfilled, your stomach likely will be, as well.

8: Swap a cup of pasta for a cup of vegetables

Just by eating less pasta or bread and more veggies, you could lose a dress or jeans size in a year. "You can spare from 100-200 calories on the off chance that you decrease the bit of starch on your plate and increment the measure of vegetables," says Cynthia Sass, RD, a representative for the Academy of Nutrition and Dietetics.

9: Always have breakfast

It appears to be a simple eating routine win: Skip breakfast and you'll get more fit. However numerous investigations show the inverse can be valid. Not having breakfast can make you hungry later, prompting a lot of snacking and voraciously consuming food at lunch and supper. To get more fit - and keep it off - consistently set aside a few minutes for a sound morning feast, similar to high-fiber grain, low-fat milk, and organic product.

10: Include fiber in your eating routine

Fiber helps processing, forestalls clogging, and brings down cholesterol - and can help with weight reduction. Most Americans get just a large portion of the fiber they need. To receive fiber's rewards, most ladies ought to get around 25 grams day by day, while men need around 38 grams - or 14 grams for each 1,000 calories. Great fiber sources incorporate oats, beans, entire grain food, nuts, and most leafy foods.

References

1. Food, Nutrition, Physical Activity, and the Prevention of Cancer: a Global Perspective. Washington DC: AICR; 2007. World Cancer Research Fund/American Institute for Cancer Research. [Google Scholar]

2. Food, Nutrition, Physical Activity, and the Prevention of Breast Cancer. Washington DC: AICR; 2010. World Cancer Research Fund/American Institute for Cancer Research. [Google Scholar]

3. Protani M, Coory M, Martin JH. Effect of obesity on survival of women with breast cancer: systematic review and meta-analysis. Breast Cancer Res Treat. 2010;123:627–35. [PubMed] [Google Scholar]

4. Clemons M, Goss P. Estrogen and the risk of breast cancer. N Engl J Med. 2001;344:276–85. [PubMed] [Google Scholar]

5. Rock CL, Flatt SW, Laughlin GA, Gold EB, Thomson CA, Natarajan L, et al. Reproductive steroid hormones and recurrence-free survival in women with a history of breast cancer. Cancer Epidemiol Biomarkers Prev. 2008;17:614–20. [PMC free article] [PubMed] [Google Scholar]

6. Verkasalo PK, Thomas HV, Appleby PN, Davey GK, Key TJ. Circulating levels of sex hormones and their relation to risk factors for breast cancer: a cross-sectional study in 1092 pre-and postmenopausal women (United Kingdom) Cancer Causes Control. 2001;12:47–59. [PubMed] [Google Scholar]

7. Goodwin PJ, Ennis M, Pritchard KI, Trudeau ME, Koo J, Madarnas Y, et al. Fasting insulin and outcome in early-stage breast cancer: results of a prospective cohort study. J Clin Oncol. 2002;20:42–51. [PubMed] [Google Scholar]

8. Kaaks R, Lukanova A. Energy balance and cancer: the role of insulin and insulin-like growth factor-I. Proc Nutr Soc. 2001;60:91–106. [PubMed] [Google Scholar]

9. Grimble RF. Inflammatory status and insulin resistance. Current Opinion Clin Nutri Metab Care. 2002;5:551–9. [PubMed] [Google Scholar]

10. Patterson RE, Rock CL, Kerr J, Natarajan L, Marshall SJ, Pakiz B, et al. Metabolism and breast cancer risk: frontiers in research and practice. J Acad Nutr Diet. 2013;113:288–96. [PMC free article] [PubMed] [Google Scholar]

11. Foster GD, Wyatt HR, Hill JO, Makris AP, Rosenbaum DL, Brill C, et al. Weight and metabolic outcomes after 2 years on a low-carbohydrate versus low-fat diet. Ann Intern Med. 2010;153:147–157. [PMC free article] [PubMed] [Google Scholar]

12. Sacks FM, Bray GA, Carey VJ, Smith SR, Ryan DH, Anton SD, et al. Comparison of weight-loss diets with different compositions of fat, protein, and carbohydrates. N Engl J Med. 2009;360:859–73. [PMC free article] [PubMed] [Google Scholar]

13. IOM. National Academy Press. Washington, DC: National Academy Press; 2002. Dietary Reference Intakes for Energy, Carbohydrate, Fiber, Fat, Fatty Acids, Cholesterol, Protein, and Amino Acids. [PubMed] [Google Scholar]

14. Eckel RH, Jakicic JM, Ard JD, de Jesus JM, Houston Miller N, Hubbard VS, et al. 2013 AHA/ACC guideline on lifestyle management to reduce cardiovascular risk: a report of the American College of Cardiology/American Heart Association Task Force on Practice Guidelines. Circulation. 2014;129:S76–99. [PubMed] [Google Scholar]

15. US Department of Agriculture. 2015–2020 Dietary Guidelines for Americans. (8th) 2015 Dec; [Google Scholar]

16. Thomson CA. Diet and breast cancer: understanding risks and benefits. Nutr Clin Prac. 2012;27:636–650. [PubMed] [Google Scholar]

17. Abete I, Astrup A, Martinez JA, Thorsdottir I, Zulet MA. Obesity and the metabolic syndrome: role of different dietary macronutrient distribution patterns and specific nutritional components on weight loss and maintenance. Nutr Rev. 2010;68:214–31. [PubMed] [Google Scholar]

18. Cornier MA, Donahoo WT, Pereira R, Gurevich I, Westergren R, Enerback S, et al. Insulin sensitivity determines the effectiveness of dietary macronutrient composition on weight loss in obese women. Obes Res. 2005;13:703–9. [PubMed] [Google Scholar]

19. Pittas AG, Das SK, Hajduk CL, Golden J, Saltzman E, Stark PC, et al. A low-glycemic load diet facilitates greater weight loss in overweight adults with high insulin secretion but not in overweight adults with low insulin secretion in the CALERIE Trial. Diabetes Care. 2005;28:2939–41. [PubMed] [Google Scholar]

20. Ros E, Nunez I, Perez-Heras A, Serra M, Gilabert R, Casals E, et al. A walnut diet improves endothelial function in hypercholesterolemic subjects: a randomized crossover trial. Circulation. 2004;109:1609–14. [PubMed] [Google Scholar]

21. Banel DK, Hu FB. Effects of walnut consumption on blood lipids and other cardiovascular risk factors: a meta-analysis and systematic review. Am J Clin Nutr. 2009;90:56–63. [PMC free article] [PubMed] [Google Scholar]

22. Rajaram S, Sabate J. Nuts, body weight and insulin resistance. Br J Nutr. 2006;96(Suppl 2):S79–86. [PubMed] [Google Scholar]

23. Sabate J, Cordero-Macintyre Z, Siapco G, Torabian S, Haddad E. Does regular walnut consumption lead to weight gain? Br J Nutr. 2005;94:859–64. [PubMed] [Google Scholar]

24. Wien MA, Sabate JM, Ikle DN, Cole SE, Kandeel FR. Almonds vs complex carbohydrates in a weight reduction program. Int J Obesity. 2003;27:1365–72. [PubMed] [Google Scholar]

25. Pelkman CL, Fishell VK, Maddox DH, Pearson TA, Mauger DT, Kris-Etherton PM. Effects of moderate-fat (from monounsaturated fat) and low-fat weight-loss diets on the serum lipid profile in overweight and obese men and women. Am J Clin Nutr. 2004;79:204–12. [PubMed] [Google Scholar]

26. Li Z, Song R, Nguyen C, Zerlin A, Karp H, Naowamondhol K, et al. Pistachio nuts reduce triglycerides and body weight by comparison to refined carbohydrate snack in obese subjects on a 12-week weight loss program. J Am Coll Nutr. 2010;29:198–203. [PubMed] [Google Scholar]

27. Foster GD, Shantz KL, Vander Veur SS, Oliver TL, Lent MR, Virus A, et al. A randomized trial of the effects of an almond-enriched, hypocaloric diet in the treatment of obesity. Am J Clin Nutr. 2012;96:249–54. [PMC free article] [PubMed] [Google Scholar]

28. Abazarfard Z, Salehi M, Keshavarzi S. The effect of almonds on anthropometric measurements and lipid profile in overweight and obese females in a weight reduction program: a randomized controlled clinical trial. J Res Med Sci. 2014;19:457–64. [PMC free article] [PubMed] [Google Scholar]

29. Shai I, Schwarzfuchs D, Henken Y, Shahar DR, Witkow S, Greenberg I, et al. Weight loss with a low-carbohydrate, Mediterranean, or low-fat diet. N Eng J Med. 2008;359:229–41. [PubMed] [Google Scholar]

30. Austel A, Ranke C, Wagner N, Gorge J, Ellrott T. Weight loss with a modified Mediterranean-type diet using fat modification: a randomized controlled trial. Eur J Clin Nutr. 2015;69:878–84. [PubMed] [Google Scholar]

31. Le T, Flatt SW, Natarajan L, Pakiz B, Quintana EL, Heath DD, et al. Effects of diet composition and insulin resistance status on plasma lipid levels in a weight loss intervention in women. J Am Heart Assoc. 2016;5:e002771. [PMC free article] [PubMed] [Google Scholar]

32. Bonora E, Targher G, Alberiche M, Bonadonna RC, Saggiani F, Zenere MB, et al. Homeostasis model assessment closely mirrors the glucose clamp technique in the assessment of insulin sensitivity: studies in subjects with various degrees of glucose

tolerance and insulin sensitivity. Diabetes Care. 2000;23:57–63. [PubMed] [Google Scholar]

33. McArdle W, K F, Katch V. Exercise Physiology: Energy, Nutrition, and Human Performance. 6th. Lippincott Williams & Wilkins; 2006. [Google Scholar]

34. Cleland CL, Hunter RF, Kee F, Cupples ME, Sallis JF, Tully MA. Validity of the global physical activity questionnaire (GPAQ) in assessing levels and change in moderate-vigorous physical activity and sedentary behaviour. BMC Public Health. 2014;14:1255. [PMC free article] [PubMed] [Google Scholar]

35. Friedewald WT, Levy RI, Fredrickson DS. Estimation of the concentration of low-density lipoprotein cholesterol in plasma, without use of the preparative ultracentrifuge. Clin Chem. 1972;18:499–502. [PubMed] [Google Scholar]

36. Abrahamson PE, Tworoger SS, Aiello EJ, Bernstein L, Ulrich CM, Gilliland FD, et al. Associations between the CYP17, CYPIB1, COMT and SHBG polymorphisms and serum sex hormones in post-menopausal breast cancer survivors. Breast Cancer Res Treat. 2007;105:45–54. [PMC free article] [PubMed] [Google Scholar]

37. Jensen MD, Ryan DH, Apovian CM, Ard JD, Comuzzie AG, Donato KA, et al. 2013 AHA/ACC/TOS guideline for the management of overweight and obesity in adults: a report of the American College of Cardiology/American Heart Association Task Force on Practice Guidelines and The Obesity Society. Circulation. 2014;129:S102–38. [PMC free article] [PubMed] [Google Scholar]

38. Look AHEAD Research Group. Pi-Sunyer X, Blackburn G, Brancati FL, Bray GA, Bright R, et al. Reduction in weight and cardiovascular disease risk factors in individuals with type 2 diabetes: one-year results of the look AHEAD trial. Diabetes Care. 2007;30:1374–83. [PMC free article] [PubMed] [Google Scholar]

39. Mattes RD, Dreher ML. Nuts and healthy body weight maintenance mechanisms. Asia Pacific J Clin Nutri. 2010;19:137–41. [PubMed] [Google Scholar]

40. Baer DJ, Gebauer SK, Novotny JA. Walnuts consumed by healthy adults provide less available energy than predicted by the Atwater factors. J Nutr. 2016;146:9–13. [PubMed] [Google Scholar]

41. Estruch R, Ros E, Salas-Salvado J, Covas MI, Corella D, Aros F, et al. Primary prevention of cardiovascular disease with a Mediterranean diet. N Engl J Med. 2013;368:1279–90. [PubMed] [Google Scholar]

42. Thomson CA, Stopeck AT, Bea JW, Cussler E, Nardi E, Frey G, et al. Changes in body weight and metabolic indexes in overweight breast cancer survivors enrolled in a

randomized trial of low-fat vs. reduced carbohydrate diets. Nutr Cancer. 2010;62:1142–52. [PubMed] [Google Scholar]

43. Thompson HJ, Sedlacek SM, Paul D, Wolfe P, McGinley JN, Playdon MC, et al. Effect of dietary patterns differing in carbohydrate and fat content on blood lipid and glucose profiles based on weight-loss success of breast-cancer survivors. Breast Cancer Res. 2012;14:R1. [PMC free article] [PubMed] [Google Scholar]

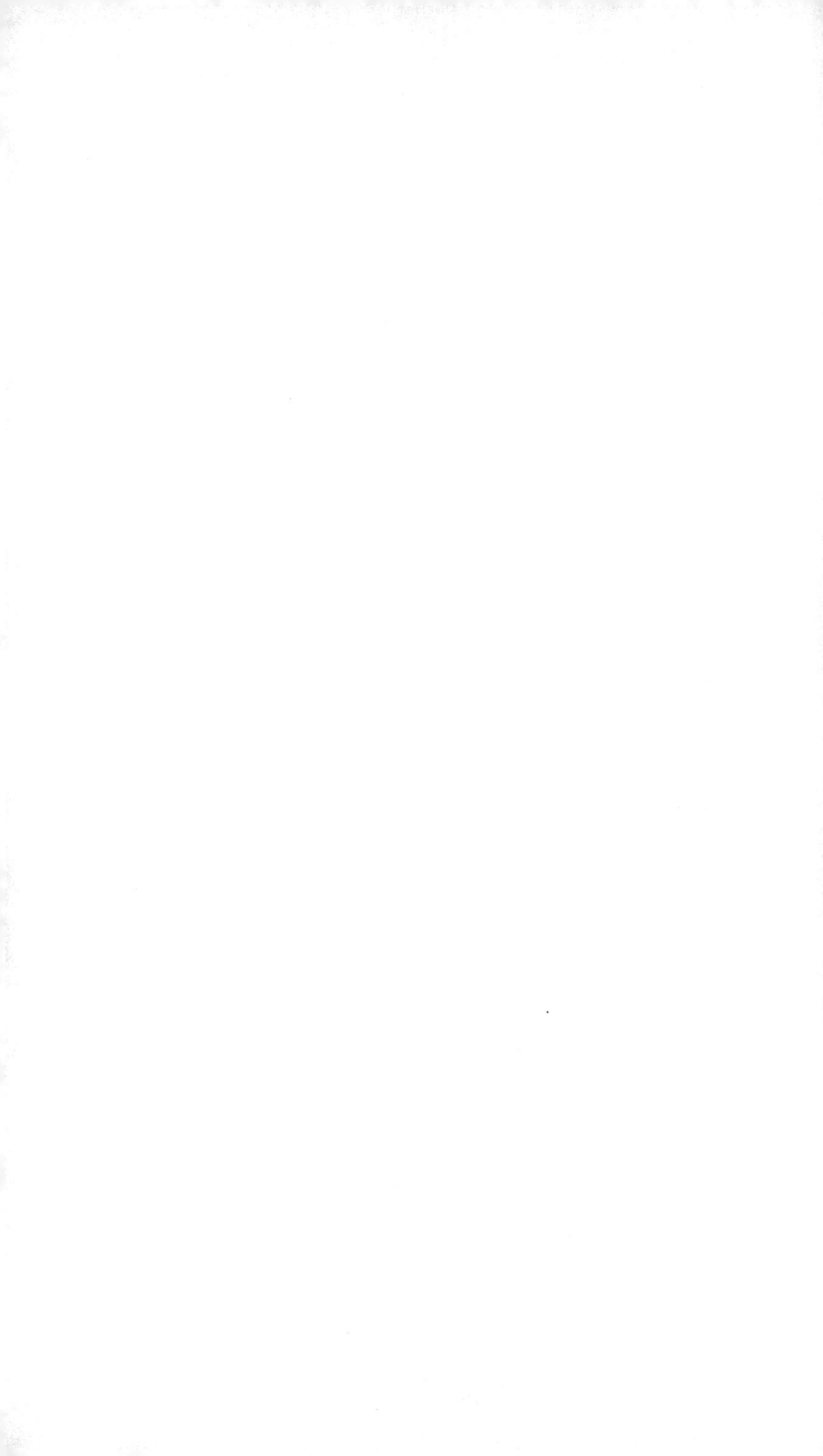